Paleo Diet Secrets

The Celebrities Diet That Works

J. Steele

**Paleo Diet Secrets Revealed
Following Miley Cyrus, Megan Fox, and Matthew
McConaughey In This Weight Loss System**

Terms and Conditions

Contents

Foreword

Those who wish to lose weight seem to have a handful of options when it comes to the diet they can try. Each diet has a particular lifestyle it is trying to promote and in order to get the best results one must adhere to it as religiously as possible.

The Paleo Diet is one of the most popular diets of today not only because a lot of famous celebrities have tried it out but more importantly because it is known to be really effective.

As compared to all the other fad diets out there, the Paleo Diet is one that is principled and based on ancient history which makes it absolutely unique. Also, this form of diet does not promote starvation or crash dieting; rather you are taught how to basically improve on your food choices to get the best results.

If you are abreast with the history, some thousands of years ago, during the Paleolithic Age, cavemen had very few options for the foods that they could eat. As a result, their food intake was usually just restricted to fish, vegetables, nuts and the like.

At the present time, advocates of this diet would basically have to adhere to the exact same principle.

We will find out about Paleo Diet here.

Chapter 1
Introduction

What This Ebook is All About

The Ebook will provide you with some of the most basic information you need to know about the Paleo Diet. You will also have a rundown of which stars are doing the diet at present and you would be surprised to know that this diet is what is making them look and feel good for a couple of years now.

Of course, you will also be taught the basic principles of the diet to ensure that you would have a clear image not only of the kinds of foods that you can eat but also the kinds of exercises you can do.

Since this diet does not require a rigorous change in your lifestyle, you are assured that you can adapt to it and it can easily change your body physically and your mind mentally.

Athletes, Executives and the Paleo Diet

This Ebook will also consist of some of the most valuable information you need to know about how athletes can benefit from this kind of diet. If you are an athlete yourself, you would immediately realize that this is the best kind of diet for you.

What's more, you will also learn that this kind of diet is ideal for those who wish to lose weight. Even those who simply want to build muscle or maintain their weight can adhere to this kind of newfound lifestyle.

If you have been searching for some ways how to lose weight effectively without gaining it all back or if you simply want to improve your strength and build your stamina, this Ebook is perfect for you.

Chances are, in no time, you would really be impressed with what all the information found in this Ebook can do for your life.

Chapter 2:
Where The Paleo Diet Came From

The Paleo Diet dates back to the principles and lifestyle some thousands of years ago. During the Paleolithic Age, cavemen were gifted with very few food options. As a result, they needed to find effective ways to survive.

Throughout the years, scientists and researchers have found that there is a huge correlation between the lifestyle of these cavemen and their resistance to various types of diseases. Thus, it is said that living the kind of lifestyle that the cavemen of that time lived would also be beneficial to those who wish to lose weight and build muscle and be more healthy.

Paleolithic Ancestors

The Paleo Diet therefore advocates the consumption of select food types that may be good for the health. Some food examples include eggs, nuts, vegetables and fish.

One may say that these food types are promoted by other types of diets out there and that may be correct. But what makes the Paleo Diet different is the fact that these food types are categorized according to their actual importance.

For instance, the basic principle of the diet is to consume the right kind of fats as long as they are natural. This means that a person advocating this diet can consume fats from animals, coconut, olives and more. The same amount of consumption is required of meats as long as they are grass-fed ruminants, pastured poultry and the like.

The consumption of vegetables is also required however it is a must that this is done in smaller amounts as compared to fats and meats. Some of the best vegetables to choose from are those that are considered to be non-starchy. As for fruits, there is only one type of fruit that can be consumed and these are berries. Lastly, starchy veggies, nuts and seeds can be consumed but only in moderation.

The Past and The Present

As mentioned earlier, the Paleo Diet dates back to the lifestyle of cavemen that lived thousands of years ago. It was during this time that various types of diseases were so uncommon and people in general lived much longer lives.

Looking into our present time and taking into account people's lifestyles today, it seems that achieving the same kind of health is quite difficult, if not absolutely impossible. With all the fast food chains lurking right outside our doorsteps, with all of the restaurants tempting us to take a bite, it is really quite difficult to achieve and eventually maintain a much improved lifestyle.

However, some people might argue by saying that this diet wouldn't work because living the lives of cavemen in present times is just impossible. If you look at the concept literally, you would surely find it difficult to adhere to. This is why those who have an open mind and those who are not afraid to try out new things for their own benefit are those that will really benefit from this kind of diet.

The Paleo Diet has changed the lives of so many people around the world. Why not let it change yours?

Chapter 3:
Foods on the Paleo Diet

A common misconception about the Paleo Diet is that it requires you to cut down on so many different food types, you would most likely be left with none.

However, one of the most important indications that a particular diet is effective is when you are still allowed to eat some of the foods that you enjoy eating but only in moderation.

Diets that require you to starve yourself for very long hours or those that require you to "crash diet" are basically those that you cannot really trust. Of course, some of the high-fat foods would really have to be eliminated from your daily meal plan because not only are these foods unhealthy, they can also trigger or cause various types of diseases.

The 80/20 Principle

The Paleo Diet greatly invests in the concept of the 80/20 diet plan. This means that you can eat certain food types 80% of the time but you should restrict yourself to eating certain foods 20% of the time.

So the question now is, how will you be able to measure whether or not you are already consuming the said percentages for foods on a daily basis?

The truth is, there is really no way of measuring this. What you can do instead is to familiarize yourself with the various food types that you can consume more of and those that you can consume in moderation. Having an idea would help guide you throughout your entire Paleo Diet journey.

Foods You Are Free to Eat

The Paleo Diet promotes the consumption of certain types of foods. Those that are found below can be consumed 80% of the time. You might feel excited to try a new diet and as a result you might want to consume these foods 100% of the time. Note that doing this is also not advisable because the body needs certain nutrition that these foods may not be able to give you.

- Leafy greens – spinach, romaine, iceberg lettuce

- Colored veggies and fruits – beets, butternut squash, spaghetti squash

- Lean meat – beef, chicken, turkey, pork, lamb, goat and the like. Make sure that you will only consume natural meats. Some fatty meats are okay as long as it's not cooked in oil

- Seafoods – shrimps, oysters, scallops, octopus, eel, fish but mackerel, salmon and tuna are your best options

- Eggs – especially raw ones. To enjoy raw eggs better, mix them with protein shakes or fruits

- Monosaturated fats and oils – olive oil, nuts, avocados, seeds, nut oils and more

- Berries – acai, strawberries, raspberries, blueberries, blackberries

Foods to Consume in Moderation

Some of the groups that you can consume but only in moderation include:

- Dark chocolate

- Alcohol – not more than a glass or two of beer or wine

- Caffeine – can only be consumed in the form of tea or coffee, not sodas

- Dairy products – cheese, milk, yogurt, butter, sour cream

Foods to Completely Avoid

- Rice

- Beans

- Potatoes

- Peanuts

- Corn

To be able to get the best results from this diet, make sure that you drink at least 8 glasses of water per day.

Chapter 4: Matthew McConaughey and The Paleo Diet

Matthew McConaughey is just one of the many famous celebrities out there who has been advocating the Paleo Diet for quite some time now.

As an actor, it is important for Matthew to keep himself fit not only to swoon the women but to also leave a good impression on those who will watch him on the big screen.

Throughout the years, it has been quite evident how the actor's body has improved tremendously and he owes this to the Paleo Diet as well as allowing him to be active most of the day. Matthew believes that it is ideal for every person to break a sweat at least once a day by engaging in an activity that can make it happen.

Although he does not always go to the gym because of schedule constraints, he makes it a point to utilize what he has at home or what he has handy to get himself fit.

Matthew's Paleo Experience

Matthew's diet is composed of consuming foods that act as the foundation of the Paleo Diet. He loves to eat high protein foods that can help build and tone muscles. What's great about his lifestyle is that there are also some instances wherein he splurges in "forbidden foods" but he knows how to make up for it the day after.

The actor is also advocating the Warrior Diet. Although not intentional, there are several instances due to his jam packed schedule that he not able to eat at the right time. Thus, he finds himself eating just a single square meal everyday which also helps maintain his lean physique.

The one-meal-per-day approach need not be a cause for alarm though. Some people may claim that this is bad because it teaches the body and the mind to starve. The truth is that, there are also several good effects to eating just one meal per day. For instance, one wouldn't feel bloated and sleeping at night is also much easier than eating with a full stomach.

Get to Know Matthew's Daily Regimen

It might come as a surprise to most people that Matthew McConaughey does not really have a concrete weight loss regimen that he does on a daily basis. Truth is that, he was able to reach his fitness goals by combining a generally healthy and active lifestyle while incorporating the Paleo Diet as much as possible.

As a result, he is able to strut a lean figure, with six packs protruding from his stomach and the most toned arms and legs in the whole universe.

You see, a change in lifestyle shouldn't be difficult especially if you are dedicated to it. What's more, incorporating the Paleo Diet into your lifestyle can also help change your life in more ways than one. And since you can eat so many different food options you wouldn't necessarily grow tired of this kind of diet. It's unique, it's effective and it is what will help make you achieve the kind of body that Matthew McConaughey has.

Chapter 5:
Megan Fox and the Paleo Diet

Megan Fox is undeniably one of the hottest and most gorgeous celebrities of her generation. As a Hollywood actress and a model, she has impressed a lot of critics and directors that immediately picked up on her talent and honed her to become better in terms of her acting and modeling career.

But this isn't really all that made Megan Fox undeniably popular. This gorgeous lady also has one of the most perfect bodies in the entire world. No wonder, she is able to easily capture the eyes of both men and women.

So what is the diet that transformed Megan's body into what it is today? It's none other than the Paleo Diet.

Megan's Relationship with the Paleo Diet

For several years now, Megan has been advocating the Paleo Diet and has been a living testimony and proof to how good and effective this diet really is.

What's great about the Paleo Diet is it's very easy to do even if it is your first time dieting so it also increases one's chances to truly change their lifestyle and lose as much weight as possible.

Even though some people might say that this diet is unhealthy because it limits the consumption of certain food types, there really is no truth to that. In fact, if you want to be able to achieve a body as beautiful as Megan's then this is the diet that you need to focus on.

Megan's Healthy Food Options

As a Paleo Dieter, Megan mostly consumes vegetables, lean meats, eggs, berries and nuts. She makes it a point to interchange the food choices so that it will never get boring. What's great to do with this kind of diet is to choose the foods you will be eating as carefully as possible because this is really what will ensure the best results.

Sample Meal Plan

If you are encouraged to try this diet for yourself because you have seen how gorgeous Megan's body looks, here's a sample meal plan that you might want to try. Of course, you can change the foods every now and then so that your palate will never get tired of tasting the same thing over and over again.

- Breakfast – Dried fruits, strawberries, grapefruit (or juice blend)
- Lunch – chicken breast, avocados, berry salad, pork loin
- Dinner – lean steak or other meats, a slice or two of salmon, mixed veggie salad

- Morning and Afternoon Snacks – almonds, pumpkin seeds, baby carrots, fresh apples

People who are doing the Paleo Diet just like Megan Fox can typically consume between 1400-1500 calories per day.

If you look at the figures closely, the amount of calories that one can consume is much higher than the calories normal people who wish to lose weight can consume on a daily basis. The figures for those who wish to lose at least 1 to 2 pounds per week should be just around 1200 calories per day.

This proves that the Paleo Diet is not only effective, it is also very satisfying and wouldn't make you feel hungry or starved at all.

Chapter 6:
Miley Cyrus and the Paleo Diet

Miley Cyrus or Destiny Hope in real life is best known for the hit show Hannah Montana where she played two characters – one as Hannah and one as herself. After a few years on television, the show was absorbed and was adapted into a movie which was also a hit especially among young children.

This is one of the biggest breaks Miley Cyrus had and after a couple more years, she gained even more popularity when she starred in a number of other movies like The Last Song and most recently, So Undercover. She is also known for having an on and off relationship with current fiancé Liam Hemsworth.

But other than all of these successes, Miley is hot in the limelight because she has transformed into one of the most beautiful actresses in Hollywood today. Not only did she cut her hair short, she also lost so much weight without having to look frail and weak. Her secret is a healthy lifestyle which consists of the Paleo Diet as well as working out regularly.

Miley's Paleo Diet Story Unleashed

Miley was actually rumored to be suffering from an eating disorder when photos of her much thinner body was posted on various websites online. To this she answered that she wasn't suffering from anything but had found a new and effective approach to losing some unwanted fat.

She started doing the Paleo Diet and immediately fell in love with the concept because she believes that it is easy to follow and does not require a rigorous process. After all, what you simply need to do is to consume the foods that are said to be good for Paleo dieters and avoid those that are considered to be "bad foods".

Other than this, Miley is also advocating a gluten-free diet that is also being promoted by the Paleo concept.

Obviously, the rumors have all gone down now because most people who have tried the Paleo Diet can easily confirm that it is indeed one of the best diets ever created and one that can provide immediate and visible results. No wonder, Miley's attire is becoming shorter and shorter which looks amazingly beautiful on her too.

Miley's Advice

Miley's advice to those who wish to lose weight? Simple! Try the Paleo Diet because not only does it help build muscles while reducing weight, it can also help improve one's skin condition along with an improved mental state. So at the end of the day, there's really nothing more you can ask for?

There are still several other Hollywood actors and actresses getting into the Paleo Diet but even if this is the case, the diet cannot be called a fad. This is because the diet is definitely here to stay especially since it provides life-long benefits and visible results no other diet can guarantee.

And since the Paleo Diet dates back to some thousands of years ago, it also helps trigger one's imagination on how it was to have lived in the Paleolithic era.

Chapter 7:
The Paleo Diet and Building Muscle

One thing's for sure: no weight loss regimen will ever work for the long run if you don't combine your cardio exercises with the best ways to build muscle.

This is primarily due to the fact that building muscle can help speed up one's metabolism making it easier to lose weight even with a little less effort.

The bottom line therefore is easy. No amount of cardio can help make you feel satisfied no matter how much sweat you expel from your body. This is because you will see visible results in your weight but your muscles will not be strengthened. This in turn becomes one of the primary causes for sagging skin especially in certain parts of the body like the arms, thighs and abdomen.

Muscle Building

It is therefore necessary to build muscles. There's no need to always lift heavy weights because doing so does not guarantee anything.

What you need is a consistent regimen that will not strain you so that you can still stick to it the day after.

This is why the Paleo Diet comes in. Since this diet is centered on changing one's lifestyle from an overall perspective, it also encourages a change in one's mindset. Basically this means that you need to not only pick yourself up and engage in any form of exercise, you also have to be wiser when it comes to your food choices.

Since the Paleo Diet is keen on promoting certain food types like nuts, dairy, berries, fish, lean meats and the like and is also demanding the exclusion of foods like rice, peanuts, fatty foods and more, it would be best to adhere to it for the best results.

At first, this new lifestyle and diet plan may seem a little difficult but just one week into it and you would immediately feel better overall.

Since you will now be consuming foods that are high in protein and low in fat, you will find it much easier to also build muscles. Of course, muscles may not be visible but if you combine this diet with the right kinds of exercises, you will definitely be able to see the huge changes in your physique.

Are there Downsides to Building Muscles?

Some people wonder whether or not there are some downsides to building muscles. Fact is, there is no downside to it. In fact, the more muscles you are able to build and strengthen the better it would be for you.

One of the indications that your muscles are growing and improving can be gauged when you can already lift heavier weights and when, no matter how often you eat foods allowed under the Paleo Diet, you still do not feel any kind of bloating or experience any weight gain.

You see, there's so much to gain with this kind of diet opportunity and since it's already right before your very eyes, it would be ideal to just go for it and see how it can change your life.

Chapter 8: The Paleo Diet and Weight Loss

A lot of people wish to lose as much weight as possible but don't really know how to go about it correctly and effectively. What's worse is that a lot of people may have tried all the diets available to them only to find out that nothing really works.

The fact is that, diets need to match your lifestyle and mindset in order for them to work. First, they should be easy to follow and they should never make you feel deprived. One diet that is keen on promoting these things is none other than the Paleo Diet.

A lot of people, along with the growing number of celebrities who are doing the Paleo Diet are most happy with it because it guarantees visible results without making you feel hungry all the time. Thus, you are able to manage your weight, gain more confidence and live a generally healthier life altogether.

How Does Paleo Diet Help in Weight Loss

First and most importantly, the Paleo Diet is centered on limiting one's food intake. With just this idea in mind, it becomes rather automatic for one to lose as much weight as possible. When this happens, the body jumpstarts and the metabolism speeds up.

At some point the body becomes used to the daily regimen so it may experience what is known as a plateau. However, with the Paleo Diet, this is something one would not necessarily experience.

The Paleo Diet limits food intake and substitutes the high-fat and 'bad foods' with healthier food options. For instance, instead of eating rice and beans, it would be best to consume vegetables and berries. Instead of drinking sodas, it would be best to drink tea. Instead of eating milk chocolates, dark chocolates can be consumed as a better substitute.

When this is done religiously, one is guaranteed to experience effective and consistent weight loss. No plateaus should be experienced and no cravings will ever be present. After all, this is just all in the mind.

Water and Weight Loss

The Paleo Diet also promotes the intake of at least eight glasses of water per day. This is to make sure that the body is hydrated properly especially if you engage in routine exercises or any other form of rigorous activities.

Also, the consumption of water is also known to have direct effects to weight loss because it helps make the body feel fuller and also helps break down stored fats. When combined with the Paleo Diet and the right kinds of exercise, weight loss goals can easily be achieved.

Is This Just Too Good to Be True?

At this point, you might think that this diet is just too good to be true but it really isn't. Some of the most famous celebrities have tried it and it has done wonders for them.

But before engaging in this kind of weight loss regimen, it is first ideal to psyche one's self to focus on weight loss goals and have an open mind when it comes to this new life-long regimen.

Chapter 9:
The Paleo Diet for Athletes

All athletes, regardless of their specific sport are required to have a healthy lifestyle in order to perform at their best. This is the very reason why most of them are particular with the kinds of diets they try because they are wise enough not to allow any fad diet to jeopardize their successful careers.

This is also the very reason why those who patronize and advocate the Paleo Diet can be trusted completely because it is guaranteed that their lives and overall health have been greatly improved thanks to this diet plan.

Rainey Wikstrom

One of the first athletes that tried the Paleo Diet is none other than Rainey Wikstrom. According to her she is a huge fan of the diet not only because it works but also because it helps her get back on track every time she relapses.

Some of the most common improvements she has experienced had to do with his physical appearance especially in certain parts of the body particularly his waist and of course her athletic performance as well.

Since Rainey won as the 2004 National Masters Athena event, she needs to continue inspiring other athletes out there not only in terms of what they can do but also in terms of what they can achieve when they try this diet. It worked for her, so it can work for anyone.

Benefits to Athletes

There are still several other athletes out there who have had the most wonderful experiences when it comes to the Paleo Diet. In fact, most of them said that they wouldn't trade this diet for anything else. It is quite surprising to hear this from athletes because unlike celebrities, they are not really one to promote any diet unless it works for them. Obviously, this one really does.

Athlete's Nutritional Requirements

Athletes who are into the Paleo Diet also need to develop the best eating habits that work for them. This includes eating the right kinds of foods before they exercise and munching on small amounts of snack foods while exercising.

Also, right after a round of exercise or training, athletes should also consume a small amount of food that can be in the form of grapefruit juice or other types of fruits like berries or apples. Of course, eating in small amounts for the next couple of hours until bedtime is also required to pump up one's adrenaline and to replenish what the body lost during the exercise.

Protein, Carbs and Fat

Every now and then, athletes who engage in serious training may bend the rules of the Paleo Diet but only up to a certain extent. Basically, this means that you can eat a few more servings of the right kinds of protein, carbs and fat because it is guaranteed that your body will be able to burn it anyway.

Of course, for best results, eating right as guided by the principles of the Paleo Diet along with exercising and living a healthy lifestyle are what's truly important.

Chapter 10: Conclusion

By now, you are probably amazed and inspired with all of the information you have read about the Paleo Diet. Hopefully you have learned valuable concepts that you can bring with you for the rest of your life.

You are now aware that the Paleo Diet is one of the best diets out there and no matter what people might say, it is still one of the most effective diets that can show you visible results. Of course, the physical changes are not the only things that should matter. More than this, you also need to be concerned about your general health.

The Paleo Diet can truly help change your life and the next thing you know, you will feel more confident about yourself like you've never felt before.

Beyond the Paleo Diet

Of course, it is normal that at some point you will start to feel tired with having to adhere to a rather strict diet. But since you know yourself better than anyone else, you will also have the ability to prevent this from happening.

A good technique when doing this diet is to change your meal plan at least twice a month so that you will never get tired of eating the same foods again and again. Also, you can create your own meals by mixing and matching various ingredients to add a wonderful taste to it.

The best mindset is to always ask yourself: "if they can do it, why can't I?" This can easily motivate you to push further and reach your goals without stopping.

Yes, a cheat day every now and then is most certainly welcomed but make sure to discipline yourself at all times. Remember your goals and stick to it – this way you will really be a good example of how wonderful the Paleo Diet truly is.

Are There Side Effects to the Paleo Diet?

If there is one diet out there that promises to not give you any problems with regards to side effects, the Paleo Diet is the one indeed.

There are no side effects with this diet. In fact, you will be gaining strength while building muscle and you will also be able to improve your overall wellbeing. As a result, you will feel happier, more fulfilled and more capable of doing things and reaching your goals at work, in school or anywhere else you might be active in.

How Much Should the Diet Cost?

There are no actual figures to determine how much the Paleo Diet would cost. Since most of the allowed foods in this diet are already available in your home, there's no need to purchase anything extra.

This diet can even help you save a huge amount of money because you wouldn't have to eat at fast food chains or restaurants that are not only unhealthy but also quite expensive.

Bear in mind that the results of this diet may differ from one person to the other and it is up to you to make yours the best result yet.

I hope that this book has given you a head start on getting started with the Paleo Diet and to have great success with your health.

Best wishes on your ventures.

OTHER RESOURCES:

Amazon Pilates Power Pack

http://scgoldmine.com/go/?aj3i

Intermittent Fasting Foundations

http://scgoldmine.com/go/?h0jo

Body Weight Blitz

http://scgoldmine.com/go/?j5fb